PREMED WORLD

PREMED WORLD

Your Journey toward Medical School

Michael Rivera-Garcia,NHA,M.P.A., M.S.H.S.

iUniverse, Inc.
Bloomington

Premed World
Your Journey toward Medical School

iUniverse books may be ordered through booksellers or by contacting:

iUniverse
1663 Liberty Drive
Bloomington, IN 47403
www.iuniverse.com
1-800-Authors (1-800-288-4677)

Because of the dynamic nature of the Internet, any web addresses or links contained in this book may have changed since publication and may no longer be valid. The views expressed in this work are solely those of the author and do not necessarily reflect the views of the publisher, and the publisher hereby disclaims any responsibility for them.

Any people depicted in stock imagery provided by Thinkstock are models, and such images are being used for illustrative purposes only.
Certain stock imagery © Thinkstock.

ISBN: 978-1-4759-3032-0 (sc)
ISBN: 978-1-4759-3033-7 (ebk)

Library of Congress Control Number: 2012909687

Printed in the United States of America

iUniverse rev. date: 05/25/2012

Your vision will become clear only when you look into your heart.
Who looks outside, dreams. Who looks inside, awakens.

—Carl Jung

The Search Within

Your eyes see a vision,
Your heart sees the truth,
Making an incision
Shows foolproof
That saving a life,
Seeing a smile,
Giving a second chance
Gives you the desire that you can enhance.
A road of discovery through knowledge and strength
Gives you the courage to comprehend that what you do and
Where you go are who you are.

—Janet R.

CONTENTS

——————▽——————

ACKNOWLEDGMENTS

First and foremost, this book would not have been accomplished without the blessing and guidance of God. Thank you for giving me health and the opportunity to gain and share knowledge with others in this project.

INTRODUCTION

I will help you analyze your career choice of studying medicine. I will also guide you and provide the best available information to enlighten your path and help you make informed decisions throughout your journey. Your first responsibility is to discover your motives for choosing this profession. The big, underrated, necessary question is determining why you want to become a doctor.

As you are reading this book, it is clear that you are very serious about entering medical school, but I would like for you to ask yourself a few questions: Why medicine? What are the forces that drive you toward this profession of becoming a doctor? Are these forces strong enough for you to dedicate your life to this profession?

As you already know, you will be faced with similar questions when you apply to medical school. These are primary questions and concerns from medical school admissions committees as well.

Take this opportunity to analyze for yourself what makes medicine so unique for you.

THE US MEDICAL SYSTEM

To become a full-fledged physician, you must understand the steps that lead to your chosen profession. This will give you a general idea about the process that prospective students must go through before they become doctors. Specific educational training and standard examinations are among the requirements for becoming a physician. My first step will be to introduce you to these.

The United States requires a lengthy series of educational steps for would-be physicians. They include undergraduate courses, medical school, and graduate medical education. I will outline the educational steps necessary to practice as a physician as well as the examination requirements:

Undergraduate Education (Four years): You will spend four years of college completing your degree in what is commonly known as a premed program. At the end of four years, in addition to any thesis work that your college requires, you will prepare for and take Medical College Admission Test (MCAT).

Medical School (Four years): The first two years consist of basic science, and the last two years consist of clinical rotations at hospitals affiliated with your medical school. Upon completion of medical school, you earn the title of Doctor of Medicine (MD). Your journey does not end here. You must enter **residency training** before being allowed to practice on your own as a physician.

There are 126 accredited medical schools in the United States. Medical schools receive their accreditation from the **Liaison Committee on Medical Education** (LCME).

Residency (3-7 years): Your chosen specialty will dictate the amount of time required to complete the residency. In general, residencies for primary care specialties, family practice, internal medicine, etc. are shorter than those for other specialties that are more invasive (surgery). This educational phase is known as **graduate medical education**. After completing medical school, you will participate in a residency program that could last between three and seven years. This professional training is conducted under the supervision of assigned physician educators. Your chosen specialty will dictate the amount of time required to complete the residency.

In the United States, there are approximately 5,000 residency programs in about 1,700 hospitals. Initial selection to a residency program is possible through the National Residency Matching Program (NMRP). Residency programs receive their accreditation from the Accreditation Council on Graduate Medical Education (ACGME).

Examination Requirements

Many books discuss the Graduate Medical Examination in great detail and offer strategies on how to pass it. Some valuable titles are listed in the resource section at the end of this book. This section is intended to give you a general idea about the examination schedules and the materials covered. These are the examination requirements that all student physicians in any medical school need to pass in order to graduate from medical school and enter into a residency.

First, students take the **United States Medical Licensing Examination (USMLE).** Every prospective physician must take this—whether they have trained in the United States or elsewhere. This evaluates a physician's readiness to enter the medical system. There are three parts to completing the USMLE:

USMLE Step 1 is a multiple-choice exam that takes approximately eight hours. It covers all the basic science courses from your first two years of medical school. The typical basic science classes are anatomy, biochemistry, physiology, statistics, behavioral science, microbiology, pharmacology, pathology, and ethics. This exam is usually taken at the end of the two years of basic sciences. Many Caribbean schools require this step in order to continue toward the clinical part of studies.

USMLE Step 2 has been divided into two parts:

USMLE 2a: Clinical Knowledge
This one-day exam covers all the clinical sciences: medicine, surgery, pediatrics, obstetrics and gynecology, psychiatry, forensics, emergency care, pathology, ophthalmology, and ethics.

USMLE 2b: Clinical Skills
Examinees are tested on their diagnostic skills. They are placed with simulated patients pretending to have complaints, and they are required to make a diagnosis based on these symptoms and other patient information.

Clinical knowledge and clinical skills are required in order to graduate from medical school and for EFCMG certification. The Educational Commission of Foreign Medical Graduates is a certificate for non-US-trained doctors that have fulfilled the requirements to practice medicine in the United States.

USMLE 3 is taken by students during their residency program within a year or so of graduation.

THE DARK SIDE OF MEDICINE

—————▼—————

Your vision will become clear only when you look into your heart.
Who looks outside, dreams; who looks inside awakens.
—Carl Jung

There are many challenges to making it through medical school. The undergraduate medical years are like a long road. It will take many years before you can practice as a physician. You will need to learn vast amounts of material faster than you were expected to during your undergraduate years. Your personal life will be consumed by more than learning and memorizing. You will also spend time with—and learn to make decisions about—sick, injured, and dying patients. As an individual you will be tested physically and emotionally to the limits of your strength.

During your residency years, you will also have the responsibility for delivering bad news to the families of those with terminal illnesses, incurable diseases, loss of life, etc. You will have long hours, depending on specialty and heavy patient load, and you will be making decisions about patient treatments. You will feel the weight of life-and-death decisions.

THE BRIGHT SIDE OF MEDICINE

—————▼—————

Many people want to become doctors to earn social status or to make a lot of money. While there is nothing wrong with these goals, they will not sustain you through the long path toward becoming a physician. A doctor's job is to help others get well; if you do not have this desire, you might not last long.

If you want to go to medical school and succeed, make this your ultimate challenge. Medicine can be a rewarding career on many levels. Medicine can also be a lucrative field after years of training. You will be involved in continuous technological advances that will aid you in helping patients. You will gain amazing knowledge about the human body. There are also intangible rewards such as the joy of helping others. You will be a major influence on your patients' health—whether concerning treatment, surgical choices, or alternative measures.

BATTLE PLAN FOR COLLEGE

———————▼———————

In war, there is no prize for runner-up.
—General Omar Bradley

There are many differences between college and high school. One of those differences is the structure on which the school curricula are built. In high school, you are more restricted in the time and classes you take; in college, you have the freedom to choose just about any major, your classes, and the time you take them.

Many new college students mishandle their freedom and end up doing things that delay their goals. Many students end up finishing their degrees later than expected or end up with a lower GPA than they need because of inappropriate planning.

Many times, it is because of a lack of guidance and structure—not because of lack of effort. Many students enter college without knowing what major they want, or they choose a major to get into college. That could help initially, but it is necessary to keep the goal in mind.

Why are you pursuing this degree? If it is a major you want to pursue to get you into medical school, do not waste your time. It is necessary to pursue a degree you like because focus without passion does not make you more successful as a student. If you enjoy what you are studying, you will put in the necessary effort to be successful because you enjoy it. If you choose a major because it will look good for medical school, it will become a drag and make it harder to be successful.

Your overall grade point average (GPA) will be evaluated, but the prerequisites carry most of the weight when you are being evaluated.

You cannot be a successful college student without proper planning. When military officers are in charge of an operation, a victory in battle is partly due to early planning. Successful tacticians like Napoleon and General Patton both had mental determination and the stamina to follow their plan to victory.

Make sure you avoid mistakes that are made by many students to ensure a successful battle plan for college.

Common mistakes include the following:

- Deciding that you do not need help. The ego is usually as major factor.
- Not seeking help early from college counselors, tutors, and department heads.
- Taking courses that are not required for your degree or medical school.
- Not seeking out a premed adviser early.
- Overloading your semester with too many courses, including too many sciences.
- Enrolling in a major that does not interest you and failing to nurture your potential.
- Committing too much time to extracurricular activities.
- Failing to set a time management plan.

Your School of Choice

For high school graduates or college students thinking of transferring to another school, picking the right college is not always easy. You don't have to go to an "A" school to be admitted to medical school. "A" schools have earned their reputation by having an excellent academic foundation, great faculty, and a sound learning environment, but they might not meet your needs for your major or as a premed student.

Survival of the fittest can be applied to the college environment. You cannot control the college environment, but you can choose the right college to meet your needs. My advice is to be a big fish in a little pond. In other words, being an outstanding student at a smaller, reputable school is better than being anonymous at a larger school. You will be able to interact more with your professors; they will have more time because they have fewer students. You will have the opportunity to ask questions that concern you, build more positive relationships with professors, and gain attention for your individual efforts. At larger universities, this is often impossible.

Why is this important? When you start applying to medical schools, you will need recommendations from professors—and possibly from your premed adviser. It is an advantage to get to know your professors. In addition to MCATs and GPAs, recommendations provide another form of evaluation for admission committee members.

State universities and private universities are sometimes more prestigious, but the prestige is often in direct proportion to the cost of tuition. According to the National Center for Education Statistics, the average cost of tuition for a private nonprofit university in 2012 was $35,000; a public university averaged $22,000.

You will almost certainly have to take out loans for medical school. Don't increase your debt by paying more than what you need to for your undergraduate work. Seek out state or private universities with a solid academic reputation—and a good premed program. At the same time, keep your eye on the price tag. While I am not disregarding the larger, more prestigious institutions, make sure you are not paying for the name as well as the education.

Be aware of the school environment. You will have a lot of work to do, and it is essential that you are in a place that is conducive to—and supportive of—your work. Lastly, keep in mind that the "big name" schools are almost always difficult to get into. If you apply to these, make sure to include some less flashy, but equally solid "safety schools."

There are a few things you should look for when looking for a college as a premed.

- Is it a four-year, degree-granting institution?
- Does it offer major you want to pursue?
- What are the graduation and retention rates?
- Does it have a premed adviser or committee?
- What types of tutoring services are available?
- What is the cost of tuition?
- What is the reputation of the university?
- Are there opportunities for volunteer clinical experience?
- How many premed students make it to medical school?

Beginning College: A Goal-Oriented Approach

Once you have chosen a college, it is time to design a road map for your goals. In order to do this, you must think and act strategically. You must think of the things that you want to do and place yourself in a position where you can accomplish those things.

Choosing a Major

"What do I like? What do I want to be studying for these four years in college? What are my strengths? And, most importantly, how can I take the premed courses through this major?"

Regardless of the major that you think will appeal most to medical school admission committees, choose a major that interests you the most. There is no favored major for medical school admissions. Typically, the vast majority of accepted college students are science majors, but this tendency is changing as medical colleges seek to diversify their student bodies. This will be your only chance to learn something else that interests you apart from medical school.

If you choose a major that interests you, your grades will likely be higher because you will put more effort into it. This is logical, but some students get so consumed with the premed protocols that they forget about what makes them happy and what interests them. Your grades in your major are as important to medical school committees as your premed courses.

Once you have you decided on a major, obtain the curriculum from the department and evaluate the program through all four years. Know the courses, prerequisites, and corequisites for each semester. It is important to understand the sequence of the courses required to obtain the degree and how the premed courses fit into your chosen major.

To Be, or Not to Be, a Science Major

If you are a science major, there will be no problem establishing the sequence of courses in the major since the premed courses are already included in most science-related majors. Courses outside of a student's major are not typically covered by financial aid unless they have been approved as an elective.

For nonscience majors, the student is responsible for scheduling his or her own premed courses. Also, for the nonscience major, the premed courses might not be covered by financial aid since they are not a requirement for degree completion. However, you might be covered if it is allowed as an elective.

Those who plan to enter—or are already in—a nonscience major should be prepared.

Since the only science courses that you will be taking are the premed courses, you will have slightly more pressure than those majoring in a science. For example, if you obtain a C in physics, your science GPA will stand out. If you have a nonscience major and end up with a poor grade in a premed course, consult your registration office. Do not waste your time; the only other chance you will have to improve your science GPA is to enroll in more advanced science courses to balance out the low premed course.

However, don't let this discourage you from majoring in economics or art history. In the past, the average applicant thought that being premed meant being a science major. This is no longer the case. Medical school committees seek students with a broad spectrum of educational backgrounds and interests.

Whether you are a nonscience major or science major, once you start taking your premedical requirements, you have already started preparing for the Medical College Admission Test (MCAT). The MCAT will be based upon the premed courses you will take in your college years. Three years of college in one exam? Impossible? No. Difficult? Yes—especially if you do not prepare.

The majority of the schools agree in their basic requirements:

- general chemistry
- organic chemistry
- general physics
- general biology

Some schools require advanced math, and a small number of schools require biochemistry. The best way to find out is through the individual websites or the Medical School Admission Requirements (MSAR) and the Osteopathic Medical College Information Booklet.

Seeking Guidance

Meet with your premed adviser while you are planning your courses. He or she can help you create a successful road map. Many students make the mistake of taking a course or courses without direction, and they end up with ineffective results. Initiate and agree upon a plan that will outline your schedule of courses—not only prior to the first semester but for the others as well. The purpose of this step is to involve your premed adviser in the process, making him or her committed to the process. The support or commitment of your counselor or adviser is vital if your strategic planning efforts are to succeed. Do your best to keep the lines of communication open between you and your adviser. He or she can direct you in planning your coursework and could even recommend professors that might fit your learning style.

Premedical advisers are there to help premeds. Do your best to get the information you need as early as possible. If you get a good adviser, do your best to keep your premed adviser informed and make appointments to update paperwork. Building a positive relationship with your premed adviser can be a good way to gain additional knowledge about the admission process and to learn about other students that have failed or succeeded at the institution. The premed adviser will get to know more about you and can provide a better recommendation when you start applying to medical schools.

Some premed advisers are very busy, poorly informed, or unable to provide the best information. On the other hand, many are student-oriented and care about student success. If your adviser says something that discourages you, do not take it personally. Advisers have seen students come and go, and their opinions come from watching others succeed or fail. You are not any of those other people. You have your chance to prove what you can do—to your adviser and to yourself. Do not give up; it just means that you have to do more researching.

Do not disregard your premed adviser because many medical schools require a recommendation from a premed adviser if one is available at your school. Most importantly, keep records of any important information you find relating to medical school. The more information you discover, the more knowledge you will have about the process. This will help you make more informed decisions.

Study Habits

> We are what we repeatedly do. Excellence is not an act but a habit.
> —Aristotle

A large part of your success in college will depend upon your study habits. A combination of discipline and routine will result in success.

Start early in your study habits. Try different methods of learning to see which one works for you. Do you study better alone or in groups? Do you learn more when you record the lectures? Do you remember better what you hear, what you see, or what you read? Do you learn more writing everything? No matter how you learn best, it is important to determine this before you go to medical school.

During college, you will have the opportunity to experiment with the methods that work best for you, gradually, without affecting your grades. Practice on your own at home. Create a home exam for a class to see how you fare in the exam. If you are not satisfied, evaluate the methods that did not work and move on to other methods. However, I suggest that you do not experiment in real class exams until you feel comfortable with your chosen method. This is your opportunity to fine-tune your learning style. Don't wait till medical school to do it; you will not have an opportunity to refine your skills because so much is demanded from you as soon as you enter. Do not expect that your study habits will change once you are accepted to medical school. Create responsible study habits and understand your learning style; the discipline and awareness will last throughout your education.

Once you have fine-tuned your skills, stick to them as if your career depended on them. It does! Maintain a routine. Most importantly, become disciplined; there is no greater enemy than lack of discipline. Make sure you can do work anytime work is required of you.

In college, all courses you take, withdraw, fail, or repeat will be recorded in your transcripts. Do not overwhelm yourself with too many classes.

Physics and Organic Chemistry

As a premed, you will take many challenging courses. However, physics and organic chemistry are by far the most feared by premed students. Do not despair; keeping yourself focused on your goal is a good way to start. These classes can be intense and challenging, but if you have a plan before you take them, it can help you to be prepared and succeed.

I initially felt overwhelmed when I took these classes; it was not till the middle of the semester that I realized I was not rationalizing each class individually. I felt overwhelmed by new words and formulas. As I began to develop strategies for these courses, I figured out my mistake. With every new chapter, I changed my game plan to adjust to the pace, shoving loose pieces of random information at my head. Finally I saw the big picture—I needed to focus on a plan and stick to it. These are general things that you need to do in order to succeed in these classes.

Organic chemistry can be intense because it is a new form of language you are not accustomed to seeing. Don't panic—anything new takes time to adjust. You may feel overwhelmed by the number of compounds, names, reactions, and mechanisms, but do not worry. You are not alone—every student that takes organic chemistry gets some type of shellshock. Your role as a student is to know the manipulation of functional groups and formations of carbon-carbon bonds; this is the basis of organic. You have to know how to make molecules react and understand what molecules make them react with each other. Organic chemistry can be a fun course, but it cannot be learned the night before the exam. Organic chemistry consists of several basic principles and many extensions of these principles.

Organic chemistry has a broad range of terminology. Try to read the major topics in the chapter before class so you won't feel lost when the professors discusses them. Check for similarities and differences in formulas and conversions. You will soon start becoming aware of the patterns in organic chemistry.

Physics can be an interesting course; it is filled with a rich history and is very challenging. Physics deals with mechanics, sound, heat, light, and electricity. In physics, you will need to focus on memorization as your primary source of study—like organic chemistry—but you will have to solve formulas with little information.

Physics must be understood. When you encounter principles and equations, analyze them and understand the equations and principles attached to it. When an equation is presented, make it a habit to connect it to its theory or principle. This can give you a better idea for approaching the equation rather than pure memorization. Memorization is good for learning the equations, but if that is the only thing you are depending on in physics, it will be a long and hard road.

Making the connections between equations and principles will make your life easier when approaching problems in physics. You will encounter difficult problems, but consider what you know about similar situations. Don't lose sight of previous equations; the approaches you used to solve those problems can be helpful as you advance from chapter to chapter.

When using memorization in physics, it is good to keep in mind that this should supplement your understanding in your approach to solving problems. When you are taking an exam and the pressure is on, your memory might fail for any number of reasons—have a way to recall information if the need arises. When trying to memorize equations, bundle them together on a sheet of paper in a logical order that makes it easier to recall.

Remember this phrase: "What do I have, and what am I missing?" This may sound straightforward and simple, but many students lose sight of this and get overwhelmed when they see so many details. Keep the same approach. Let's break this phrase down:

What do I have? These should be the first objective. What is the problem presented giving me? Is it force and mass? If it is, then this is what I have to work with. Put these items aside and ask what things have been given to me in the problem that can help me resolve this problem.

What am I missing? Recall the equations that were given to you in class discussions or in the chapter. Once you are clear with what you have, relate them to the equations that might fit the description to the problem you are solving. Look at examples of similar problems in the assigned chapters.

In summary, for physics and organic chemistry, you need to practice daily, read actively, listen, work out problems, and reread and reorganize your notes.

Faculty Interviews

I interviewed Dr. Charlene McWhinney and Dr. Maria Plummer, associate professors at New York Institute of Technology.

Organic chemistry has always been a course that premed students have always been concerned about when enrolling. What mindset or approach should students take in these courses?

CM: Understanding chemistry will help the student appreciate the chemistry in the human body. Chemistry is the basis of all biology.

MP: I think that may students approach organic chemistry and similar courses with unfounded trepidation and see it as a "rite of passage" to medical school. I may have done so myself. Rather, it's a good opportunity to assimilate a large body of material and learn how to organize one's time and manage a difficult subject area. This is good training for the medical school curriculum. At times, it may seem that the connection between organic chemistry and clinical medicine is not always relevant—and that may be frustrating to the premed student—but there are important links, especially in regards to pharmacology, and their efforts will be rewarded.

Many students that enroll in these courses fail the course or end up with deficient grades. From your experience, what do you see as common mistakes that undergraduates make that hurt their chances of excelling in this course?

CM: Both organic chemistry and physics require the student to learn new material and to understand it. I think that most students do not put enough effort into these courses. Also, practicing homework problems is essential for passing exams.

MP: Again, I think it's time management and organization. Being overwhelmed is very easy if you don't stay on top of the material. As in medical school, many of these courses have a lot of material presented per lecture or lab period. It's important that the student review notes every night and not wait for the weekend or before exams like he or she might for less intense courses.

Also, visual aids may be helpful. Charts, graphs, and models (especially in organic chemistry) may be useful for some students. I also like index cards because they're portable and you can bring them with you anywhere. The material may be difficult, but it's not insurmountable as long as time and energy is put into preparing for lectures and reviewing material. If a student really doesn't understand some concept or topic, pride needs to be put aside, and he or she needs to seek assistance from the professor.

Many students state that pure memorization will help any student excel in this course. Others feel that understanding is more important. What advice can you give students on this issue?

CM: Both courses require an understanding of the materials to be able to apply the information to word problems. Each course does, however, require some memorization of facts.

MP: I really don't believe in pure memorization per se, although I have used this method. In some cases, it's the only thing that can work. Memorization is effective in things such as learning the charges of chemical ions, the names and structures of amino acids, certain chemical and physical formulas, certain biochemical pathways, etc. There is just no way around those things. But, in general, even after a student memorizes something, it will stay put longer if he or she understands the concept well. One can sometimes figure out a formula if you understand the concept behind a formula, for example, cardiac output = stroke volume x heart rate. If someone knows that an element needs to be stable under a certain condition, then he or she knows that NaCl (sodium chloride) has to be Na+ and Cl—and *not* Na+2 and Cl-, which would be written Na2Cl and doesn't exist. So I think that understanding is much more important than memorization. A student can get by and even do pretty well with memorization, but in the long run, understanding is what really counts.

Survival Tips for College Classes

There are essential things to remember in order to be successful in your premed classes. As you encounter these courses, here are some things that might be helpful for surviving and improving yourself during college:

- Focus on the subjects discussed in class. These are the things your professor wants you to learn.
- Rewrite your notes from class at home; you will relearn the material.
- Do not overwhelm yourself trying to learn everything at once.
- Do not fall behind. Practice whenever possible.
- If you feel yourself being overwhelmed, ask for help. Schools usually have good tutors. Talk to academic advising or your premed adviser to help you find a tutor.
- Use the knowledge of the professor whenever possible. Ask questions during class or after class.
- If you find a compatible classmate to study with, try it. This will only be effective if you can learn and share knowledge. This is only recommended once in a while; you need time to practice the problems on your own.
- If you think the textbook is not a good book, there are always supplemental books that can help you. You can find these books in a bookstore, or you can try to find used ones from other students.
- Do not cram; study for a few hours every day. Don't study for five hours at a time; this is counterproductive. Allow yourself breaks and relax. Study smart—not hard. If you study a few hours every day, you can practice the problems from that day and still have time to review topics for the next day. This will keep you up to date—you will be able to ask good questions or provide answers.
- Check to see if the school has any resources that you can use to practice.
- If you find yourself stuck, review similar problems on the same topic.
- Finally, there is no substitute for practice, practice, and practice.

Getting the Best from a Tutor

Whether you're having difficulty with a single subject or many subjects, a tutor can be another tool you can use during difficult classes. A school tutor or a graduate tutor can be a great source of information, guidance, and motivation. Many students feel they don't need a tutor because tutoring is a waste of time. Every student can benefit from tutoring sessions—whether they utilize them once or many times.

Tutors have been through those classes and can show you the techniques they used and others have used to solve specific problems. If you're lucky, tutors might know the professor and tell you how best to approach the class.

As a former tutor, I believe that many students do not take full advantage of tutoring services. Not knowing how to take full advantage of a tutor can hurt a student's ability to obtain a higher grade.

Common mistakes I have witnessed include

- not identifying trouble signs early;
- an inability to decipher material effectively; and
- a desire to be taught again.

Not Identifying Trouble Signs

Most of us, during our college years, have had trouble mastering a subject (or subjects). However, that doesn't mean we cannot succeed in learning it. The problem becomes serious when we fail to realize that help is needed. Whether it is physics, organic chemistry, or any other course, it is important to realize when you're having continual difficulty with approaching a specific problem or concept. Seek help early if you see you are becoming confused about a problem or concept that is a part of the material under discussion.

Many students do not know they have a problem until they get a test back with a failing grade. Once this occurs, many students become frustrated and end up failing or getting lower grades than expected. This doesn't have to happen to you.

An Inability to Decipher Material Effectively

The professor sets the tone for what he or she wants students to learn from chapter to chapter. The topics, techniques, and concepts that your professor brings up in class will naturally be the ones he or she wants you to focus on.

Students often make the mistake of not prioritizing what's important, leading them to try to study everything at once. I've had students say, "The professor discussed Chapter 7 and 8; can you explain them for me?"

I always advise my students that this is the wrong approach to succeeding in these classes. It is practically impossible for a tutor to discuss all the concepts from two chapters and still maintain the same pace of the class. Tutoring sessions are limited; the best way a tutor can help you is when you are having trouble with specific problems. This enhances the effectiveness of the session since you are prioritizing what you need to learn.

In order to optimize your time with a tutor, your approach should be as follows.

- Have specific problems available—the ones you're having the most problems with.
- Work through the problem at home first—this enhances the effectiveness of the session and helps you prioritize what you need to learn.

Since the tutor will not always know what the professor has emphasized, it is your job to pay attention in class and target those problems for attack with your tutor. The best students work this way, and it is good practice for medical school.

Tutor, Teach Me Again!

There is a clear difference between going to class and seeking help from a tutor. Failing to realize the difference can block your chances of having an effective tutoring session. The role of the professor is to teach the material on the subject matter. The role of the tutor is to guide you in your understanding, to improve your ability to dissect, and to help solve the individual problems.

It seems natural to give the problems to the tutor and let him or her solve them or explain them to you. The problem is given to the tutor, the tutor solves the problem, he or she explains the problem, and then you go home. When you try to solve the problem later, you don't even know where to start.

Instead of learning by doing the problems yourself, you're trying to learn by watching someone else do them. This won't work; you may understand the solution process while your tutor is explaining it, but you won't be able to retain it or apply it to other problems.

The 50-50 Relationship

The right approach is what I refer to as the 50-50 relationship. This is the ideal relationship to have with your tutor. The student and tutor will each put forth 50 percent of the effort. It is clearly not enough to show up to a tutoring session and just watch. You need to be engaged and make sure that the session works for you.

Getting the most of your tutoring session begins with knowing what it is you expect.

- Try the problems at home first—this is your opportunity to go through the thought process on your own, and it's an important part of understanding the material. Once you have tried the problems, even if you couldn't complete them, you can go to the tutor and receive the guidance you need to complete the problem.

- Make an appointment after you have tried the problem(s). Many times, students are anxious to see their tutors and the problems have not been attempted prior to the session.

Summertime

For most students, summer is the most anticipated season of the year. For premed students, this time gives you the opportunity to seek opportunities separate from academics. Extracurricular activities are important because they can improve your profile for medical school.

Medical schools want to know what you have done to back up the reasons you have for going to medical school. Have you worked or volunteered in a health care environment where medical care is administered? Getting medical experience should be your first priority when deciding what extracurricular activities to involve yourself in.

Hospitals and clinics are good places to volunteer to get a first look at a medical work environment. Volunteer in a department that you believe you want to be involved in when you practice medicine. For example, if you always desired to work with infants then volunteer in the pediatric environment. This experience will not only help you get a firsthand look at medical care—it will also give you an opportunity to see if pediatrics is what you really want. Don't go into it with the mindset of it being a burden; look at it as an opportunity to gain more knowledge and help you plan your future career as a physician. Your experiences will also give you more to say when the interviews come.

Extracurricular activities that are not related to medicine are fine. You can also involve yourself in activities that interest you as a person. If you choose this route, make sure that your activity is unique to your premed counterparts. Don't do something that you do not like; involve yourself in an activity that is unique to your character and that you enjoy. If you have doubts about what activities you could get involved in during your free time, consult your premed adviser. They can provide guidance and give you an idea about previous students' activities. This information can help you to stay away from activities that are commonly undertaken by premedical students. You need to be different and competitive to gain an edge over other applicants. Medical school committees want to know if you are a well-rounded student.

Extracurricular activities play an important role in student applications, but these activities should never come before your academics. Your grades are very important, and extracurricular activities will not excuse poor grades. Make sure that your activities do not overwhelm you and do not take time away from your studies. Some schools offer summer internships in related fields, usually at the student center.

MCAT

The Medical College Admission Test is a requirement for entry into almost all American medical schools. The MCAT is a standardized, multiple-choice examination created to assess problem-solving, critical thinking, and writing skills. It is another way to objectively evaluate student performance in relation to other students.

Many students argue that a B in an elite school equals an A in a small liberal arts college. They believe that the weight of the school will bring them closer to medical school; this might not be far from the truth, but it does not guarantee entrance. Remember that a B is what it is—no matter where you got it. It is preferable to be a big fish in a small pond than a small fish in a big pond. An A in any accredited four-year university is what it is.

Medical school admissions staffs cannot judge the prestige of a school while evaluating a student's academic performance. The MCAT brings balance to the equation. The MCAT is an objective form of measuring a student's performance and stamina.

The MCAT is administered twice a year; it should be taken no later than April of the year of application. If you take the August MCAT, you will be at a disadvantage for some schools. You have to wait approximately sixty days to receive your scores, which will delay your application process. Your application will not be processed without it being complete.

Be aware that some medical schools have rolling admissions. In those cases, applications are reviewed as they are received.

The MCAT consists of

- physical sciences (physics and general chemistry);
- biological science (biology and organic chemistry);
- verbal reasoning; and
- writing samples.

The physical sciences section consists of eleven passages on physics and inorganic chemistry. In physics and general chemistry, you will be dealing with graphs and tables and learning to integrate problems to solve them.

The biological sciences section consists of eleven passages on biology and organic chemistry. This is based on solving problems, integrating concepts, and analyzing tables and graphs. For the MCAT, it is not enough to memorize—although it can be helpful. It is impossible to know exactly which problems you will get.

The last two parts of the MCAT are not scientifically based, but they are no less important. Take these two sections as seriously as the science ones. A high score in the sciences will not compensate for low scores here. Admission committees want students that can read, interpret, and communicate.

The verbal reasoning section consists of nine passages. Reading passages, magazines, newspapers, and any other form of lengthy literature can stimulate your reading comprehension.

You will be given two essay questions. Take an English composition course; it is not only helpful—it is necessary. You will learn to produce the thesis of your arguments, develop paragraphs, and develop concluding statements.

Preparation for the MCAT

The MCAT should be taken as seriously as your premed classes. Do not listen to your premed classmates that say you do not have to prepare much for this exam. Do not think that your preparation for the MCAT should be minimal because you are doing well in the premed courses. You need to prepare for it.

You do not need any advanced science courses to take the MCAT. It will be no good if your GPA is great, but your MCAT is not. There are many guides and tips for how to prepare for the MCAT. There is no secret formula to pass the MCAT; you have to study hard with the right materials. Your effort and your commitment to this exam will reflect how badly you want to get in. It will take a lot to prepare and study for this exam; always keep focused on the reasons you need good scores.

It is never too early to start preparing for the exam. The average studying time is four months; it should be no less than two months. Eventually you will have to choose a route of study to prepare for the test. Depending on your learning style and other factors, you can choose between precourses or self-study for the MCAT.

Commercial Courses or Self-Study?

Commercial courses can be quite expensive. Many students have mixed feelings about taking commercial precourses. They agree that the material received was worth it. In commercial courses, you have the opportunity to take timed practice exams, which can be helpful for improving your stamina. You also receive feedback on your weak areas. When considering a commercial course, ask yourself the following questions.

- Do I have the money to enroll in the course?
- Do I have the time to commit?
- Do I need to be pressured to study?
- Do I need a structured environment to simulate my learning routine?

Self-study can work if you can simulate your own study environment with self-discipline, your own practice exams, and your own practice scores. You can purchase commercial course materials from students that have previously taken them. Do what works best for you. Everyone has their own learning style; some need to be pushed, and others do not. When considering the self-study route, ask yourself the following questions.

- Can I create a plan of study on my own?
- Can I become a disciplined self-learner for this test?
- Can I provide my own feedback?

Many students ask whether they should go back to their old notes from classes and start from there. I believe this is counterproductive because the overwhelming sorting of material can lead to studying unnecessary material. You lose precious time deciding what is important and what is necessary. If your choice is self-study, purchase material that has already been deciphered for you by experienced authors. There are plenty of quality materials to help you study for the MCAT.

The following companies provide courses for preparing for the MCAT. You can purchase their study material. This is the best material in the market.

- Kaplan
  www.kaplan.com
  1-800kaptest
- Princeton Review
  www.princetonreview.com
  1-800-2Review
- Exam Crackers
  www.examcrackers.com
  1-888-krackem

These materials will help you refresh, improve, and gain additional knowledge with tips, approaches, and material for the MCAT, but this is not sufficient if it is not applied to practice exams.

Whichever route you choose, practice is the ultimate requirement for success on this test. The best source for the most accurate practice test is AAMC (www.aamc.org/students/mcat/start.htm). You can find the hard-copy practice tests. Do not take the MCAT without purchasing these practice tests. These previously administered MCAT tests will give you a taste of what to expect. You can also find the MCAT student manual, which will provide more in-depth information on how to prepare for each section of the exam.

University: SUNY College Student
Interview: Stephen Fryer
Interviewer: Michael

MCAT Scores:
13PS 6VR 12BS S
Overall Score: 31S

What was the study method you used?
Practice, practice, practice.

Which practice materials did you use?
AAMC practice materials were used for all three sections and are the only practice problems. The practice problems in the AAMC are the most accurate representation of the current MCAT. I also used a Kaplan study guide.

How long did you study for the MCAT?
I studied over a four-month period, just taking practice exams. I have other friends who studied for shorter periods, but I felt I needed more time.

Taking practice tests and practicing with conditions similar to the real thing will help condition you for the exam. If you have a hard time staying focused while reading on your own, I recommend the course. If you are disciplined, save your money and purchase the review books.

Some of my friends who took the courses did very well. Ultimately, it depends on you. Do you feel you need a structured environment and a classroom setting to force you to study, or can you fall into your own routine?

Overall, my advice is to create a plan where you write down how much time you will dedicate to studying—and you stick to it. If you can do that, you will be successful! Don't give up!

Application Budget

Before you start applying to medical school, you will need sufficient funds for the MCAT, American College Application Service (AMCAS), and secondary applications. Budgeting is a process that must be tailored to each individual. You either have sufficient income—or you do not. If you are like most college students that depend on part-time jobs or students loans, creating a budget mindset early is definitely important.

Developing a money management mindset might not be the most important factor you might have to deal with during your process toward medical school, but not having one can hurt your plans. Make yourself responsible and project the amount of money you will need when it is time to apply.

There should be a direct relationship between what you expect to have and the expenses you expect. Decide on the number of schools you want to apply to early. This will give you an accurate amount that you need when it is time to apply. Do not wait for last minute to scramble for your money. Design a plan that will help you get the money you need beforehand.

Identifying Medical Schools

Identifying potential schools can be a difficult task. There are many medical schools that you can apply to, but you must narrow it down to the schools that fit your needs. Your first task will be to research medical schools in your state. Begin with in-state schools because most in-state schools give preference to their residents. Use the Internet or your local bookstore to research medical school admission requirements, *Barron's Medical School Guide*, or call schools to obtain their brochures.

> As you obtain this information, do not forget to look at the average GPA of previous classes, the average MCAT scores of previous students, the ratio between students who applied and students who were accepted, and the ratio between accepted in-state residents and out-of-state applicants.

Conduct detailed research for each school.

- Curriculum: Find out how the curriculum is based. For example, how many days and hours are you in class? How is the system of grading? Is it by letter grades or pass and fail? Pass and fail alleviates some pressure for students who have plenty of daily pressures.
- Career path: Is the school geared toward primary career teaching or research?
- Clinical: How are your clinics? Where you conduct them is very important. The location of your clinical will determine the experience you will receive.
- Environment: Consider the location of the school.
- Overall Cost: No matter what school you go to, the cost of medical school education has risen. Do not worry—when you complete your degree, you will make enough money to pay back the loans. If you have a choice of two medical schools that you consider equal and one of them is a state school, choose the state school. These schools are less expensive and provide a quality education.

Applying to Medical School

When you finally complete the prerequisites and the MCAT, you can begin to apply to medical schools. To apply to medical school, you will need to use AMCAS. For the few schools that are not members of AMCAS, you will have to apply to them directly.

AMCAS is a nonprofit, centralized application processing service for applicants to the first-year entering classes at participating American medical schools. They process, evaluate, and forward your evaluation to the medical schools you have chosen. They are neutral in the sense that they have no decision-making power in the process of individual medical schools, but they are no less important in the process.

www.aamc.org/students/amcas/start.htm
Association of American medical colleges (AAMC)
2450 N Street NW
Washington DC 20037-1123

AMCAS permits you to fill out one application that can be used for all the schools. When you complete your application, you will be required to submit your transcripts from all schools attended and your MCAT scores.

You will be asked for your fees for each school you apply to. Until recently, it was $150 for the first application and $50 for subsequent applications. This can add up, depending on the number of schools you apply to. Most students apply to ten or twelve schools—your odds increase with each application.

When you receive your secondary applications from the schools you applied to, you will be asked for an additional application processing fee that could range from $50-100.

There are several things to remember when submitting your primary application to AMCAS.

- Transcripts should be your priority. Many previous students have made the mistake of leaving transcripts for the end since all they have to do is request them. Do not make this mistake because your AMCAS application will be put on hold until your transcripts are received. Request your transcripts early so you can give time for AMCAS to evaluate them.
- Know which schools you want to apply to before you start the application. If you know the amount of schools you want to apply to, you will not delay your application and will be able to know any expenses sooner.

Letters of Recommendation

Applying to medical school is competitive, and many applicants have similar credentials in terms of GPA and MCAT scores. A few good recommendations can boost your application. Medical school committees want to see those recommendations come to life. The professor should be able to describe characteristics about you in more than one dimension—and not only about your academics.

Although it is good if a professor can indicate that you are at the top of your class, it should say something about you in the recommendation. Here is an example of my personal recommendation given to me by a professor I admire and respect.

> Date
> Office of Admissions
> Address and name of school
>
> To whom it may concern:
>
> It is my great pleasure to recommend Michael Rivera for admission to the graduate program at _____ University. Michael's potential for success in research and graduate school is excellent.
>
> Michael is an intelligent, highly motivated, and diligent student whose academic performance is outstanding. I have come to know Michael in my position as a professor and academic adviser at _____ College. Here he serves as a peer tutor in biology and chemistry, generously giving his time and knowledge to his fellow students.
>
> Michael is personable, caring, and respectful. I would be both pleased and proud to follow his career and would encourage you to look favorably on his application.
>
> Professor's Name
> Title

I have included this recommendation so you can evaluate its dimensions. This should be the type of recommendation you want for yourself—not for what is says, but for what it contains. Take a closer look, and you can see how it comes to life. You get to know more about the person than merely academics.

In the following, I provide the dimensions that were present in the previously posted recommendation. These are the dimensions that generally should be in a recommendation:

Academics:
Academic performance is outstanding.
Potential:
Michael's potential for success in research and graduate school is excellent.
Character:
Michael is personable, caring, and respectful.
Motivating Factors for Admissions:
Michael is intelligent, highly motivated, and diligent.

You want your professor to not only to talk about you being the top 5 percent of your class—but also about other dimensions that the medical school committee might not know. Medical school committees want to learn more about you and how others perceive your character and how that could be linked to medicine. Medical school committees want to know if you are the right candidate.

Getting a recommendation from a professor that knows you well enough in all these dimensions can give you an edge. It can be the difference between you and another applicant with similar credentials. It can add strength to your application or reinforce it. Your recommendation does not to have to include all dimensions. The people that you seek a recommendation from should know you in all these areas in order to provide a complete evaluation. You do not want a mediocre recommendation—you want it to stand out and come to life.

When asking people for a recommendation, make sure you ask in a graceful manner if they think they can provide a recommendation that can get you into medical school. If they indicate that they do not have enough information about you to provide a stellar recommendation, thank them and continue your search.

Strategic Alternatives

Premed students often make the mistake of reassuring themselves that they will get accepted to the medical school of their choice. For many students, the sad truth rains upon them when they receive their rejection letters. No premed is immune to such threats of rejection, but having contingency plans can help you stay on course.

Sometimes a picnic is ruined by rain, but that does not mean you will not eat. The same goes for medical school. Receiving a rejection letter from medical school does not mean you won't reach your goals—it just means it has been somewhat delayed. Contingency plans are necessary for these situations.

What contingency plans should I have in place for a worst-case scenario like being rejected from medical school?

Reapplying

If you are patient and really want to go to an American medical school, reapply the following year. You can arrange with medical schools to find out your weak areas and any other items they might have found deficient. Once you locate your weak areas, work on them. If you scored low on the MCAT, retake it. If your science GPA was low, find out about post-bachelor's premed programs in your state. Also, talk to you school adviser and discuss your options.

   The second, and most important, option is to diversify yourself. You will need to expand your application outreach. You will need to increase the number of applications submitted to medical schools. Also, combine your applications with Doctor of Osteopathy (DO) schools to increase your chances of being accepted to medical school.

Foreign Medical School

If you decide that reapplying to an American medical school just isn't in your plans, then all is not lost. You can still fulfill your dreams of becoming a physician by going to a foreign medical school, specifically in the Caribbean.

Physician Assistant

If you feel that you still do not want to reapply and do not want to go to a foreign medical school and still want to practice medicine, a physician assistant program would probably best suit your needs.

The person who cures is not always an MD. The MD is not the only option for you to gain clinical knowledge in medicine, treat the sick, and be part of continuous medical advances. Other health care professions provide direct care to patients, treat, counsel, and prescribe medications when necessary.

Doctor of Osteopathic Medicine

DO's are fully qualified physicians. They are licensed to perform surgery and prescribe medication in all fifty states. They require a four-year medical education as allopathic physicians. They can practice in a specialty area as MDs, and they also pass comparable state licensing exams.

The content of osteopathic education is the same as that of MD medical schools except that osteopaths have additional class hours devoted to osteopathic manipulation. They bring a little extra to medicine in which they practice a holistic approach for the "whole person." They receive extra training in the muscular skeletal system. This training helps them better understand how an illness can affect the body as a whole. Osteopathic physicians have the same practicing privileges in all states as their MD colleagues.

You might not have heard of a DO because few schools producing them. Becoming a DO is becoming a physician. Whether you are DO or an MD, you are a physician. If you have the passion to become a physician, this is a good career choice.

The application process is similar to becoming an MD. You must plan early. If you are able to plan your economic budget early, you might have the opportunity to apply to an MD and DO school. The DO applications are similar to the MD programs, but they are not administered by AMCAS.

AACOM
http://www.aacom.org/
5550 Friendship Blvd., Suite 310
Chevy Chase, MD 20815-7321.

Physician Assistant

This great career choice holds the future of health care delivery. In business, competition is based on the principles of microeconomics; prices, quality, and services are determined by supply and demand in the marketplace.

American medical care is becoming more and more competitive; administrators are forced to contain costs from within. Budget constraints and limits in funds have forced changes in the service delivery of our hospitals. Hospitals are forced to make internal changes for their survival. Producing quality services at a lower cost is the business point of view in any industry.

How can hospitals continue to provide efficient and effective services to patients at a lower cost to hospital payrolls? Physician assistants are at the forefront of these changes. They are medical professionals who can treat, diagnose and follow up as well as their MD counterparts. Second, they provide a higher flexibility to hospital payrolls. A starting salary for a primary physician in a primary care specialty can be $160,000. The average salary for a PA is around $63,000. Note: This stated average salary can vary from state to state.

By no means am I stating that MD's or DO's are in danger of employment. My point is to demonstrate the importance of PA's in the health care community—not only for patients but for hospitals. In the future, we will see PA's playing a larger role in our health care system.

Employment of PA's is expected to grow much faster than the average for all occupations through the year 2012 due to the anticipated expansion of the health services industry and an emphasis on cost containment, resulting in increasing utilization of PAs by physicians and healthcare institutions (Bureau of Labor Statistics, US Department of Labor, 2004).

Physician assistants are health care professionals licensed to practice medicine with physician supervision. They conduct physical exams, diagnose and treat illnesses, and order and interpret tests. In many states, they can write prescriptions. PA's can prescribe medications in at least forty-seven states. If you want to learn about the programs and careers as a PA, you can find it in the following sites:

Educational Programs:
Association of Physician Assistant Programs
950 North Washington Street
Alexandria, VA 22314-1552.
http://www.apap.org

Careers as a Physician Assistant:
American Academy of Physician Assistants Information Center
950 North Washington Street
Alexandria, VA 22314-1552.
http://www.aapa.org

Interview with a Physician Assistant

Milly Rivera
B.S. Psychology, B.S. Physician Assistant Studies
Hospital for Special Surgery, New York

Before PA school, what career, educational, and/or personal choices made you decide to go into the physician assistant profession?

I had never heard of the PA profession until my second year at Long Island University. I met a fellow student who was applying for the program. I was informed that it is a profession to practice medicine with certain liberties and certain restrictions.

The PA profession has a rich history and has become more in demand than ever before. In your own words, what would you say the PA profession is and what is so unique about it?

The PA professional is the "alternative MD." It's the practitioner who follows the medical model as a physician would. The same principles, regulations, and philosophy are incorporated within the medical education received by this breed of practitioners. PA's are unique in the sense that they share about the same information as physicians and practice with the same ideals.

Many students reading this book would be curious to know if you feel you have missed out on something by not going to medical school.

I feel that I have not missed out on going to medical school because I have about the same experience as physicians (attend medical conferences, continued medical education (CME); prescribe meds, history and physicals, perform procedures within our scope of practice), and all this accomplished within a shorter time span than medical school.

Working under a doctor's supervision, do you feel at any time restricted toward your practice in medicine?

Actually, "physician supervision" is a broad term. Physicians can supervise you in many forms without actually being physically present (making themselves available through pages, cell phones, or interacting via online services). The restriction, I believe, is your responsibility to the patient. Practice medicine in a professional, knowledgeable manner that will further enhance the profession and give the utmost care to the patient.

How do you view the future of the PA profession from your experience?

It is a rapidly growing field that deserves much attention due to its great participation in medicine. Overall, it is a career that continues to be in demand and will continue to grow.

What advice can you provide students who intend to become PAs?

My advice would be to continue forward because the studies alone require a lot of time, dedication, and self-discipline. In general, the studies require two years of prerequisites (basic sciences) and two years of professional phase (after acceptance into the program). There are also licensing and registration requirements.

Seeking employment, especially right after graduation, requires some effort, but this can apply to any field. It takes determination. Eventually you will be hired and gain the experience that will help you grow and prosper. It is educationally competitive, clinically rewarding, economically satisfying, and highly in demand.

FOREIGN MEDICAL SCHOOLS

▼

A pessimist sees the difficulty in every opportunity;
an optimist sees the opportunity in every difficulty.
—Sir Winston Churchill

What would make you consider a foreign medical school? First, international medical schools geared toward American citizens provide an opportunity for nontraditional applicants and those who might not have been chosen to study in the United States. Not being accepted to an American medical school program does not necessarily mean you are not fit to become an MD. Many qualified applicants do not get accepted because of the limited number of spots in American medical schools.

There are many reasons why students go overseas to study medicine—not everyone goes because he or she was rejected from an American school. Some students have applied first to foreign medical schools because they do not want to wait the mandated year. Older students with advanced degrees don't want to waste a year waiting a year to begin the program. Foreign schools allow you to apply and start courses the same year. Some want to start immediately, especially nontraditional applicants who have degrees in other areas and realize that medicine was their calling all along. In some, if not all, Caribbean medical schools, you can know in less than two months if you were accepted after submitting all appropriate documentation. You can also start that same year. For whatever reason students choose foreign medical schools, the decision should be evaluated carefully.

Caribbean Medical School Evolution

During the 1980s and 1990s, attending a foreign medical school was a concern for many professionals and critics. Mexico, the Dominican Republic, and the Caribbean were destinations for many Americans. During these periods, studies demonstrated major deficiencies in these schools. The conclusion was that these schools were in no way comparable to the American medical system. The concern was that prospective students studying medicine abroad were investing time and money on a substandard education. These foreign schools were mostly criticized because of their admission requirements, facilities, equipment, faculty, and curriculum.

A few schools providing medical education in the Caribbean were geared for American citizens. These schools were lacking the necessary resources to improve, expand, and restructure themselves. In the 1990s, a major overhaul commenced and the applications to medical schools were high. Many students that were qualified were unable to obtain entrance. As a result, many students began to seek alternate routes to obtain their medical degrees outside the United States.

Caribbean medical schools began to increase in number, changing the market arena for older, more established schools. Some schools have gone through changes that have changed them into credible schools for studying medicine.

As more medical schools in the Caribbean opened their doors, it changed the environment for other medical schools in the Caribbean. The influx of new schools in the Caribbean influenced, changed, and promoted competition. The increased competition in the marketplace was advocated by economists. This increased competition made clear to these Caribbean schools that changes were imminent. In management terms, these organizations were facing external threats to their survival—and those changes needed to be addressed. This stimulated some schools to formulate strategic plans to ensure the survival of their institutions.

Caribbean medical schools needed to create strategies in response to these strategic issues. They changed their marketing agenda, internal infrastructures, and recruitment of full-time faculty and support staff. As a result, some Caribbean medical schools are now credible learning institutions for their host country and the United States. They have improved facilities, financial packages, housing accommodations, standards of admissions, and professors. Most importantly, the restructuring of curriculums became comparable to the American medical system.

Not all schools in the Caribbean deserve such positive remarks since they are far from being an appropriate choice for studying medicine. It is important to research the schools you are interested in. Familiarize yourself with all aspects of each school you might be interested in.

Going to a foreign medical school can be difficult for any student, but it can provide you an alternative route to becoming a physician.

Physician Interview

Palay Srinivasan, MD, is a primary care physician in Orlando, Florida.

What is your specialty?

I am a family practice physician.

It is important to have clinical experience. How important is it to shadow a physician or clinical exposure?

It is important to get a feel for what the medical profession is all about before one would make a decision about pursuing a medical career. It also helps one to make a decision whether one would like to be a provider at all or choose a different career. But it is not mandatory if one is eagerly seeking a career in medicine.

Many students want to know what habits they should start creating as a premed and beyond. How were you successful as a premed? Any specific habits would recommend for students?

One has to stay dedicated and focused toward final goal. Hard work is the key to success. Make friends with students who are competitive and challenging. Don't start a family or relationship until you reach residency since you will have not much personal time. Have hobbies to wear down work stress.

It is understood that there are thousands of applicants per medical school application. The reality is that many students might not make the cut the first time around or even at all. If a student does not get accepted into medical school, what do you think are viable options?

Pursue a career in areas like pharmacology, microbiology, nursing, or allied health professions. Allied health professionals include nuclear medicine/CT/MRI/ultrasound/X-ray technologist, respiratory technologist, physical therapist, pharmacist, medical technologist, nurse practitioner, and physician assistant. Of course, they are challenging careers and may give you opportunities to work with patients.

What is your opinion of foreign medical schools?

Only few countries send talented doctors to America. India, Pakistan, the Philippines, Colombia, and Nigeria are worth mentioning. I am proud to say that India sends many talented physicians to different parts of the world. These foreign physicians are willing to work hard and can easily fit into American work culture.

You surely have worked alongside these two different professions. What is your opinion on the PA profession and NP profession as an option?

Physician assistants can work only under the supervision of a physician. In other words, they cannot work alone. But a nurse practitioner can work like an independent provider and can bill insurance. Simply put, it is better to be nurse practitioner than physician assistant.

What can you tell a student who is interested in medical school?

Aim higher and be dedicated in order to be successful in medicine. Honesty and integrity are prerequisites for the medical profession. Don't just think about money; you have to like the profession. You should know how to balance professional and personal lives in order to be successful in both.

Judging Foreign Medical Schools

Choosing the right medical school is an important step in determining a quality education and the ability to practice in the United States.

When choosing a school in the Caribbean, you must choose wisely because it can mean the difference between practicing medicine and not. There are many factors to consider when choosing a medical school. One of the most important factors that should come into play is your objective analysis. It is important that you stay focused on what is important.

Do not judge a Caribbean medical school by its external environment. It is important to note that a school should not be judged on conditions that are beyond its control. Food costs, currency rate, weather conditions, island conditions, and other external environmental scenarios are beyond the school's control. The conditions on any of these islands are below the standard of living in the United States.

For the most part, the economy is overwhelming agricultural. Sugar is the principal pillar. Standards of living are low in many parts of the Caribbean, especially in the agricultural islands with high populations. However, the essentials are always available.

Is the school financially and educationally committed to its students? Has the school invested in equipment and facilities? Has the school improved, added, or restructured its curriculum, enhanced access of literature, and provided other services to help students prepare for the USMLE? Internal environmental factors can be controlled by the school; it is a good sign if the school is committed to benefit students with long-range planning.

General Requirements

Even before you start doing research on medical schools in the Caribbean, they must meet the following general requirements in order to obtain licensure in the United States:

- Be listed in the World Directory of Medical Schools
- Be listed in the International Medical Education Directory (IMED)
- Obtain an ECFMG certificate
- Have a curriculum comparable to the American medical education system that is no shorter than thirty-two weeks

The World Health Organization is the United Nations specialized agency for health. Their objective is for all people to attain the highest level of health. They are responsible for publishing a list of all medical schools worldwide. The school of interest must be listed in the World Directory of Medical Schools published by the World Health Organization. www.who.int/entity/en

International Medical Education Directory (IMED)

IMED provides current and accurate information on international medical schools and their recognition that has been confirmed by the host country of the medical school. Schools operating on any island in the Caribbean must be granted legal rights by the government to grant medical degrees.

International Medical Education Directory
c/o FAIMER
3624 Market St., 4th Floor
Philadelphia, PA 19104
USA

ECFMG
The Educational Commission for Foreign Medical Graduates (ECFMG) is a prelicensing process that evaluates the readiness of international school graduates to enter accredited residency programs in the United States.

www.ecfmg.org
3624 Market Street
Philadelphia, Pennsylvania
19104-2685

Evaluating Specific Schools

Searching for the right school does not have to be a painful process, and your school most definitely should not be chosen by a gut feeling. Look beyond short-term solutions and plan for the future. Your goal is to become a doctor. If you have chosen to go to a foreign medical school, by no means should it be a substandard education.

As a premed student, you will sacrifice, study long hours, miss get-togethers, and be unable to go out on some weekends—do not settle. You are working hard to become a good physician, and you deserve and want to receive a quality education, so you should not settle for a second-rate education. Choosing the right medical school is in your hands. There are no shortcuts through medical school. Special arrangements in the curriculum beyond those that are comparable to the traditional American medical school system are unacceptable.

Apart from the school being listed as WHO-, IMED-, and ECFMG-eligible, there are specific things you want to know before you put your final stamp of approval on the school of your choice.

- *Track Record.* Do not judge a school based upon how long it has been established. Consider USMLE pass rates, clinical experience, and residency appointments since the time of establishment.
- *USMLE Preparation.* When researching schools, USMLE preparation does not necessarily mean if the school endorses a commercial prep course. If this is the case, then that is a bonus. The methods used in the curriculum assist in providing further development in preparation for the USMLE. Does the school have final exams similar in structure to the USMLE? Does the school culminate its basic science at the end with an internal review session?
- *Licensure.* Obtaining licensure to practice medicine is by far one the most important criteria of all others. Make sure that the school you choose is approved to be licensed in the state that you wish to practice. What will all those years of training and sacrifice be for if you cannot practice medicine in your chosen state? You can ask the school and verify the information with your state medical boards.
- *ACGME*(Accreditation Council for Graduate Medical Education). Caribbean medical schools have an edge over other foreign schools for those seeking licensure in the United States because you can perform many—if not all—of your clinicals in the United States. When evaluating a Caribbean school, ensure that the clinical rotations that you will be performing are ACGME approved. Many states require that the core rotations be done in ACGME-approved hospitals in order to get licensed.

Please note: Each state will and can enforce standards and requirements they deem appropriate to ensure competency.

The Department of Education and Foreign Medical Schools

Students attending foreign schools are eligible for loans under the Federal Family Education Loan Program (FFELP), but only three Caribbean schools participate in it. This program is comprised of subsidized and unsubsidized loans. Subsidized loans are provided to students who have demonstrated financial need, and the government pays the interest while the student is in school. The unsubsidized loans are provided to students regardless of financial need, but the government will not pay the interest.

The Department of Education has always been committed to help qualified students reach their goals of higher education. In the fiscal year 2000-2001, it was estimated that there were more than 13,000 students studying abroad, and 9,000 were medical students. Many of these students received federal loans. This number is important since it means that millions of federal dollars are being sent overseas to institutions of higher education to provide education to American citizens abroad. Ultimately the government is responsible for its handling of funds to these schools.

Financial Aspects:

There are several elements that determine a foreign school's ability to receive federal loans.

- Does the school have loans?
- Are they Stafford Loans?
- Is it only dependent on alternative loans?

In the Caribbean, only St. George's Medical School, Ross Medical School, and American University of the Caribbean (AUC) have been granted authority to use Stafford Loans for their students. These are good because they are mainly dependent on your financial need and American citizenship. On the other hand, these loans may not be sufficient because they might only cover tuition—and you also need living and personal expenses. You might need to request alternative loans, which are credit based. Most Caribbean medical schools use med achiever loans or TERI Loans.

These alternative loans are based on credit? It is important to verify your credit to ensure your ability to request loans for tuition coverage. Many people need cosigners for loans. Request a copy of your credit report from all three credit reporting agencies since discrepancies can exist between reports. This can help you view you report and verify and correct any mistakes on your credit report that you need to clear up before you apply for financial aid. Do not wait to get rejected from your loan to verify your credit. This can delay your entrance date. Do not let this happen to you—plan early.

You can verify your credit with the three credit bureaus:
www.equifax.com (800) 685-1111
www.experian.com (800)311-4769
www.tuc.com (800) 916-8800

If you want to order all three reports at once you can go to:
www.qspace.com

Personal Income

How much you need to save before going to a foreign medical school depends on the financial package awarded to you and when your loans get disbursed to you. Always try to save as much as you can without leaving any debt behind that might hurt you in the long run. You have to apply for your loans during your years of study.

Do not permit an old debt to haunt you—pay off everything before you leave. Once that is done, verify the cost of living on the island. Once you have done this, do not leave without your first month's expenses. If the average housing expenses are between $400-500, take $700. If you spend $300 in food per month, take $500. Do not forget the first semester books that you have to buy. Ask the school if there are any other fees that you should know about.

Some loans do not get disbursed until you are already enrolled, which leaves you with nothing until that comes through. There is one particular school in the Caribbean that requires you to pay the first semester's tuition before they reimburse you.

Foreign medical graduates are less alienated than they once were, but the alienation has not disappeared. There have been attempts to slow down the flow of foreign medical graduates to the United States, but foreign medical graduates are still permitted in the United States. It is a good time for future foreign medical graduates to gain entrance to practice in the United States.

Foreign medical graduates have filled many gaps in areas that once were considered underserved by practicing physicians. Foreign medical graduates practice next to American medical graduates. Some major hospitals have accepted foreign medical graduates because they have a credible reputation for being competent and resourceful. The normal selection process includes the following:

MD: US Medical Graduates
DO: Doctor of Osteopath
MD: Foreign Medical Graduate (US Citizen)
MD: Foreign Medical Graduate (J-Visa, Non-US Citizen)

If you decide to go to a foreign medical school, verify that the school has clinicals in the United States. Call the school directly. Are American clinicals restricted? Will you have to coordinate your own clinical? Will you have to do clinical anywhere else? Can you perform your clinical in one state? Are the hospitals ACGME-approved?

Calling Home

One thing that gets overlooked by students is researching different forms of communication for those going overseas. It is easy to get consumed by the preparations for going overseas only to realize you want to call home once you are there. Many students buy expensive calling cards, making it costly and inconvenient. There are several different ways to communicate with loved ones back home.

These are the most common:

- landline phones;
- cell phones; and
- calling cards.

All of these are available in any country, but determine the most cost-efficient way to do it. The most popular of the products is Internet phone service. Their pricing packages are the most affordable of the three. Students have reported that Vonage and Skype are the most reliable services to use. For Internet phone service, you need to have a high-speed connection.

Becoming a physician takes time, endurance, and desire. The health care system is dynamic. As a physician, you will be part of remarkable scientific and clinical advances.

As a physician, your knowledge, advice, and guidance will be sought by others. You will learn valuable lessons in communication, time management, patience, and kindness.

Whether you are going overseas or to another state, maintain your support systems. Support systems are family and friends who you can discuss your daily events with. Going through medical school will make you face many things you have never been challenged with; communication is therapeutic.

Being away from home can be challenging because your family network is not present. You might miss your routine; many students have trouble coping with such dramatic changes. It is important to note that family and friends play a huge part in your emotional well-being. The stresses in this career require immediate support. As humans, establishing, creating, and maintaining relationships is what we do. The absence of such factors can lead to mood decline, depression, and the potential loss of drive. These issues can be overlooked during applications, interviews, studying, etc.

What can we do to prevent the feeling of isolation?

- Start collecting e-mails, phone numbers, and addresses from the people you want to stay in contact with. Don't forget to give out yours if you have not already done so.
- If you had a hobby back home, continue that routine. You do not want to stop everything you did because that adds a lot of strain. Your hobbies help you release stress.
- Research phone services before you depart.

If you really want to know what it is like to become a doctor, I recommend a video of real doctors in medical school. This is by far the best video I have seen related to this topic. If you still have VHS, I urge you to see it. The company is called WGBH Educational Foundation and the video is provided by Nova. Here is a brief description of the video:

MD: *The Making of a Doctor*

Description: This is a reality-based video that goes behind the scenes of real emergency rooms and hospitals with seven students trying to become doctors. It follows a group of Harvard students throughout the rigors and rewards of their medical training. It shows you the intensity and what it does to these students as they prove themselves as future practitioners.

- You view them during their grueling academic training during basic science.
- You view them during their clinical (usually second and third year).
- You view them during their residency.

Although it was made around 1995, it is still a video you must see.
Rating: 4 out of 4
You can also check out *Survivor MD* from Nova. To order from Nova, contact:
WGBH Video
P.O. Box 2284
South Burlington, VT 05407-2284

Step 1: www.wgbh.org.
Step 2: Go to Shop
Step 3: Product Search, Title of Video References:

Textbooks should be your primary source of study, but many textbooks have a few problems. No student should take organic chemistry and physics without buying the solutions manual for the assigned textbook. You will get more opportunity to practice and start understanding the patterns involved with each topic. If you have additional time and would like additional help, supplemental books are always a good choice.

RESOURCES

———————▽———————

Organic Chemistry 1& 2, General Physics 1& 2.
1—REA'S problem Solvers: Complete Solution to all textbooks
Research and Education Association
61 Ethel Road West
Piscataway, New Jersey 08854
www.rea.com

This book provides detailed examples of problems and solutions. This is intended as a supplement to your textbook—not as a replacement. This book is divided in thirty-five chapters, covering every topic you might encounter in organic chemistry.

FINAL NOTE

Always put your patients first—and service their physical, psychological, and emotional needs whenever possible. Realize medicine is a rationalistic science, and some diseases are terminal, but paramount to this philosophy is to lessen human suffering whenever possible through existing and experimental treatments. However, remember that you do not treat a fever chart or a cancerous growth, but a sick human being whose illness may affect the person's family and economic stability.

As you enter medical school and go on to practice medicine, remember the positive forces that drove you to this profession. Do not permit the two most important letters that you have worked so hard in your career to become M and D (Money-Driven).

In conclusion, do your best to put humanity first. Always remember that medicine is one of the oldest and most revered professions. Do your best to honor it.

Thank you.

Michael Rivera, MPA

> It is not your aptitude, but your attitude,
> that determines your altitude.
> —Zig Ziglar

Printed in the United States
By Bookmasters